The Essential

GASTROPARESIS COOKBOOK

for Beginners

Habeeb Ganiu

Dedication

To everyone who is cooking their way to a better and healthier life.

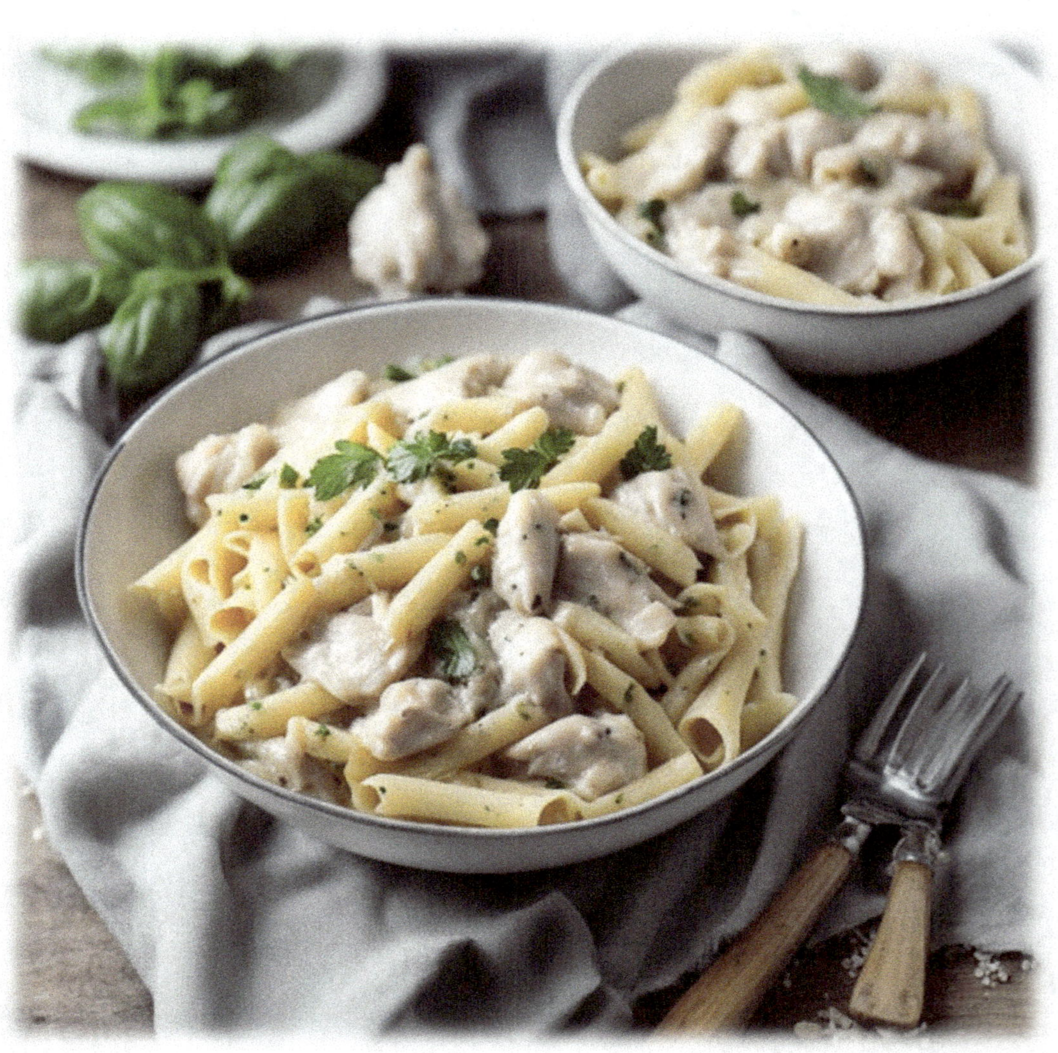

Table of Contents

Introduction

When I was first diagnosed with gastroparesis, I felt overwhelmed and lost. The simple act of eating, which once brought joy and comfort, had become a source of anxiety and pain. I struggled to find foods that my body could tolerate, and the lack of resources available to help guide me through this journey was disheartening. It was through trial and error, countless hours of research, and a lot of perseverance that I began to piece together a dietary plan that worked for me.

This cookbook is the culmination of that journey. My hope is that it will serve as a beacon for those who are facing similar challenges. I understand the frustration and fear that can come with a gastroparesis diagnosis, but I also know that with the right tools and knowledge, it is possible to manage this condition and lead a fulfilling life.

The recipes in this book have been crafted with care, keeping in mind the specific needs of those with gastroparesis. They are designed to be gentle on the stomach while still being flavorful and satisfying. I have included a variety of options to suit different tastes and dietary preferences, whether you are looking for something light and refreshing or hearty and comforting.

Beyond the recipes, I have included sections on nutrition basics, meal planning, and cooking techniques. These are the strategies that have helped me the most, and I believe they can make a significant difference for you as well. My aim is to provide not just a collection of recipes, but a comprehensive guide that supports you in every aspect of managing your diet.

Gastroparesis can feel isolating, but you are not alone. This book is a testament to the fact that there is hope and there are ways to regain control over your eating and your health. I am deeply grateful for the support of my family, friends, and medical professionals who have helped me along the way. It is my greatest wish that this cookbook will be a source of comfort, encouragement, and practical help for you.

Chapter 1: Before You Get Started

Understanding Gastroparesis

Definition and Explanation of Gastroparesis

Gastroparesis is a chronic condition characterized by delayed gastric emptying, which means that the stomach takes longer than normal to empty its contents into the small intestine. This delay occurs without any physical blockage, but rather due to the improper functioning of the stomach muscles or the nerves that control them.

In a healthy digestive system, the stomach muscles contract to move food into the small intestine for further digestion. However, in individuals with gastroparesis, these contractions are weak or uncoordinated, leading to the retention of food in the stomach. This can result in various gastrointestinal symptoms and nutritional deficiencies, significantly impacting a person's quality of life.

Symptoms and Diagnosis

Symptoms

The symptoms of gastroparesis can vary in severity and may include:

- **Nausea and Vomiting:** These are among the most common symptoms. Vomiting may occur several hours after eating, as the stomach struggles to empty its contents.
- **Bloating and Abdominal Pain:** Patients often experience a feeling of fullness and discomfort in the abdomen, even after eating small meals.
- **Early Satiety:** This is the sensation of feeling full after eating only a small amount of food, which can lead to inadequate caloric intake.
- **Heartburn and Gastroesophageal Reflux:** Delayed gastric emptying can cause stomach acid to back up into the esophagus, leading to heartburn and acid reflux.
- **Changes in Blood Sugar Levels:** Gastroparesis can affect the timing of food absorption, leading to erratic blood sugar levels, which is particularly concerning for people with diabetes.
- **Loss of Appetite and Weight Loss:** Due to the discomfort and nausea associated with eating, individuals may lose their appetite and consequently lose weight.

Diagnosis

Diagnosing gastroparesis involves a combination of medical history, physical examination, and specific diagnostic tests. Here are the primary methods used:

- **Medical History and Physical Examination:** The doctor will take a detailed medical history, asking about symptoms, their duration, and any underlying conditions, such as diabetes. A physical examination will help to rule out other potential causes of the symptoms.
- **Gastric Emptying Study (GES):** This is the most definitive test for diagnosing gastroparesis. The patient consumes a meal containing a small amount of radioactive material, and imaging is used to track the rate at which food leaves the stomach. A delay in gastric emptying confirms the diagnosis.
- **Upper Gastrointestinal (GI) Endoscopy:** This procedure involves inserting a thin, flexible tube with a camera down the throat to examine the stomach and small intestine. It helps to rule out any physical obstructions that could cause similar symptoms.
- **Ultrasound:** An abdominal ultrasound can help to exclude other conditions such as gallbladder disease or pancreatitis.
- **Gastric Emptying Breath Test:** This non-invasive test measures the rate of digestion by analyzing the breath after consuming a meal tagged with a non-radioactive isotope.
- **SmartPill:** This is a capsule that, when swallowed, transmits data about the digestive tract's pH, temperature, and pressure as it travels through the stomach and intestines, providing information on gastric emptying time.

The Role of Diet

Diet plays a crucial role in managing gastroparesis. Since the stomach's ability to process and empty food is impaired, choosing the right foods and meal patterns can significantly alleviate symptoms and improve quality of life. Proper dietary management can help in:

- Reducing symptoms such as nausea, vomiting, bloating, and pain.

- Ensuring adequate nutrition and preventing malnutrition.

- Stabilizing blood sugar levels, particularly important for those with diabetes.

- Maintaining a healthy weight.

Foods to Avoid

Certain foods can aggravate gastroparesis symptoms and should be limited or avoided:

- **High-Fiber Foods:** Foods high in fiber can be difficult to digest and may cause bezoars (hardened masses in the stomach). Avoid raw vegetables, fruits with skins and seeds, whole grains, and legumes.
- **High-Fat Foods:** Fatty foods can slow gastric emptying and worsen symptoms. Limit fried foods, fatty cuts of meat, full-fat dairy products, and heavy cream.
- **Carbonated Beverages:** These can cause bloating and discomfort due to the gas they release.
- **Alcohol and Caffeine:** Both can irritate the stomach lining and exacerbate symptoms.

Foods to Include

Focusing on easily digestible, low-fiber, and low-fat foods can help manage gastroparesis symptoms:

- **Lean Proteins:** Chicken, turkey, fish, eggs, and tofu.
- **Refined Grains:** White rice, plain pasta, white bread, and low-fiber cereals.

- **Cooked Vegetables:** Carrots, zucchini, squash, and potatoes (without skins).
- **Canned or Cooked Fruits:** Applesauce, canned peaches, and pears without skins.
- **Low-Fat Dairy:** Skim milk, low-fat yogurt, and cheese.
- **Soups and Broths:** Homemade or low-sodium commercial options that are blended or strained.

Supplements and Their Role

For some individuals with gastroparesis, maintaining adequate nutrition through diet alone can be challenging. Supplements may be necessary to fill nutritional gaps:

- **Multivitamins:** To ensure adequate intake of essential vitamins and minerals.
- **Protein Supplements:** Protein powders or liquid protein supplements can help meet protein needs.
- **Electrolyte Solutions:** Helpful in maintaining electrolyte balance, especially if vomiting is frequent.

Tips for Eating and Drinking

- **Small, Frequent Meals:** Eating smaller amounts more frequently can help manage symptoms better than larger meals.
- **Chew Thoroughly:** Thoroughly chewing food can aid in digestion.
- **Stay Upright:** Remaining upright for at least an hour after eating can help facilitate gastric emptying.
- **Hydrate:** Drink fluids throughout the day, but not too much during meals to avoid feeling overly full.

By understanding these nutrition basics, you can create a dietary plan that helps manage gastroparesis symptoms while ensuring you receive the necessary nutrients for overall health.

Sample Meal Plans for Different Stages of Gastroparesis

Gastroparesis can vary in severity, and dietary needs may change over time. Here are sample meal plans for different stages:

Stage 1: Liquid and Pureed Diet

During this stage, focus on smooth, easy-to-digest foods that are liquid or pureed to help manage symptoms and avoid exacerbating the condition.

Breakfast: Vanilla Pudding (Chapter 7: Desserts)

Snack: Chia Seed Pudding (Chapter 7: Desserts)

Lunch: Smoothie Pops (Chapter 6: Snacks and Small Bites)

Snack: Lemon Sorbet (Chapter 7: Desserts)

Dinner: Berry Compote (Chapter 7: Desserts)

Stage 2: Soft and Blended Foods

At this stage, incorporate soft and blended foods that are gentle on the stomach while still providing necessary nutrients.

Breakfast: Greek Yogurt Parfait (Chapter 3: Breakfast Recipes)

Snack: Banana Ice Cream (Chapter 7: Desserts)

Lunch: Baked Apples (Chapter 7: Desserts)

Snack: Chocolate Avocado Mousse (Chapter 7: Desserts)

Dinner: Pumpkin Custard (Chapter 7: Desserts)

Stage 3: Soft Solids

Soft solid foods can now be included, and it's important to chew food thoroughly and eat small, frequent meals.

Breakfast: Rice Cakes with Avocado (Chapter 3: Breakfast Recipes)

Snack: Baked Sweet Potato Fries (Chapter 6: Snacks and Small Bites)

Lunch: Hummus and Veggie Sticks (Chapter 6: Snacks and Small Bites)

Snack: Apple Slices with Almond Butter (Chapter 6: Snacks and Small Bites)

Dinner: Mini Quiche Cups (Chapter 6: Snacks and Small Bites)

Stage 4: Maintenance Diet

Transition to a maintenance diet with well-tolerated, nutrient-dense foods. Continue to focus on small, frequent meals and chew food thoroughly.

Breakfast: Greek Yogurt Parfait

Snack: Cucumber Bites with Cream Cheese

Lunch: Caprese Skewers

Snack: Blueberry Crumble

Dinner: Rice Pudding

Chapter 2: Breakfast Recipes

Banana Smoothie

Servings: 2

Cooking Time: 5 minutes

Ingredients

- 2 ripe bananas
- 1 cup low-fat yogurt
- 1 cup skim milk
- 1 tablespoon honey
- 1/2 teaspoon vanilla extract

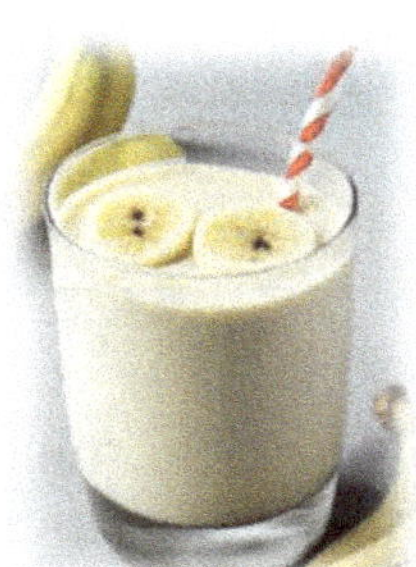

Instructions

1. Peel the bananas and cut them into chunks.

2. Place all ingredients in a blender.

3. Blend until smooth.

4. Pour into glasses and serve immediately.

Nutritional Values (per serving):

- Calories: 210 • Protein: 8g • Carbohydrates: 42g • Fat: 2g • Fiber: 2g

Soft Scrambled Eggs

Servings: 2

Cooking Time: 10 minutes

Ingredients:

- 4 eggs
- 1/4 cup skim milk
- 1/2 teaspoon salt
- 1 tablespoon butter

Instructions

1. Whisk eggs, milk, and salt together in a bowl.

2. Heat butter in a non-stick pan over low heat.

3. Pour the egg mixture into the pan.

4. Stir gently until eggs are just set and creamy.

5. Serve immediately.

Nutritional Values (per serving):

• Calories: 180 • Protein: 12g • Carbohydrates: 2g • Fat: 14g • Fiber: 0g

Applesauce Oatmeal

Servings: 2

Cooking Time: 10 minutes

Ingredients

- 1 cup rolled oats
- 2 cups water
- 1/2 cup unsweetened applesauce
- 1 tablespoon honey
- 1/2 teaspoon cinnamon

Instructions

1. Bring water to a boil in a saucepan.

2. Stir in oats and reduce heat to a simmer.

3. Cook for 5 minutes, stirring occasionally.

4. Stir in applesauce, honey, and cinnamon.

5. Serve warm.

Nutritional Values (per serving):

• Calories: 190 • Protein: 5g • Carbohydrates: 40g • Fat: 3g • Fiber: 4g

Cottage Cheese with Peaches

Servings: 2

Cooking Time: 5 minutes

Ingredients:

- 1 cup low-fat cottage cheese
- 1 cup canned peaches, drained and diced

Instructions

1. Divide cottage cheese between two bowls.

2. Top each serving with diced peaches.

3. Serve immediately.

Nutritional Values (per serving):

- Calories: 150 • Protein: 14g • Carbohydrates: 18g • Fat: 3g • Fiber: 2g

Creamy Rice Pudding

Servings: 4

Cooking Time: 20 minutes

Ingredients

- 1/2 cup white rice
- 2 cups skim milk
- 1/4 cup sugar
- 1 teaspoon vanilla extract
- 1/4 teaspoon ground cinnamon

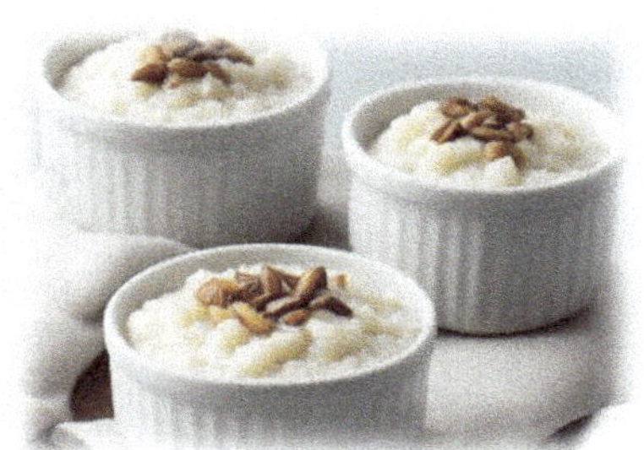

Instructions

1. Cook rice according to package instructions.
2. In a saucepan, combine cooked rice, milk, and sugar.
3. Cook over medium heat, stirring frequently, until thick and creamy (about 15 minutes).
4. Stir in vanilla extract and cinnamon.
5. Serve warm or chilled.

Nutritional Values (per serving):

- Calories: 150 • Protein: 4g • Carbohydrates: 30g • Fat: 2g • Fiber: 0g

Blended Fruit Yogurt

Servings: 2

Cooking Time: 5 minutes

Ingredients

- 1 cup low-fat yogurt
- 1/2 cup canned fruit cocktail, drained
- 1 tablespoon honey

Instructions

1. Place all ingredients in a blender.

2. Blend until smooth.

3. Pour into bowls and serve immediately.

Nutritional Values (per serving):

• Calories: 130 • Protein: 6g • Carbohydrates: 25g • Fat: 2g • Fiber: 1g

Egg White Omelet

Servings: 2

Cooking Time: 10 minutes

Ingredients

- 4 egg whites
- 1/4 cup skim milk
- 1/4 teaspoon salt
- 1 tablespoon chopped chives
- 1 tablespoon olive oil

Instructions:

1. Whisk egg whites, milk, salt, and chives together in a bowl.

2. Heat olive oil in a non-stick pan over medium heat.

3. Pour the egg mixture into the pan.

4. Cook until eggs are set, folding the omelet in half.

5. Serve immediately.

Nutritional Values (per serving):

• Calories: 80 • Protein: 10g • Carbohydrates: 2g • Fat: 3g • Fiber: 0g

Berry Smoothie Bowl

Servings: 2

Cooking Time: 10 minutes

Ingredients

- 1 cup frozen mixed berries
- 1 cup low-fat yogurt
- 1/2 cup skim milk
- 1 tablespoon honey
- 1/2 teaspoon vanilla extract

Instructions:

1. Place all ingredients in a blender.

2. Blend until smooth.

3. Pour into bowls and serve immediately.

Nutritional Values (per serving):

• Calories: 160 • Protein: 7g • Carbohydrates: 32g • Fat: 2g • Fiber: 4g

Peach Smoothie

Servings: 2

Cooking Time: 5 minutes

Ingredients

- 1 cup canned peaches, drained
- 1 cup low-fat yogurt
- 1/2 cup skim milk
- 1 tablespoon honey

Instructions

1. Place all ingredients in a blender.
2. Blend until smooth.
3. Pour into glasses and serve immediately.

Nutritional Values (per serving):

• Calories: 140 • Protein: 6g • Carbohydrates: 28g • Fat: 2g • Fiber: 1g

Vanilla Rice Pudding

Servings: 4

Cooking Time: 25 minutes

Ingredients:

- 1/2 cup white rice
- 2 cups skim milk
- 1/4 cup sugar
- 1 teaspoon vanilla extract

Instructions:

1. Cook rice according to package instructions.
2. In a saucepan, combine cooked rice, milk, and sugar.
3. Cook over medium heat, stirring frequently, until thick and creamy (about 20 minutes).
4. Stir in vanilla extract.
5. Serve warm or chilled.

Nutritional Values (per serving):

• Calories: 150 • Protein: 4g • Carbohydrates: 30g • Fat: 2g • Fiber: 0g

Baked Apple with Cinnamon

Servings: 2

Cooking Time: 20 minutes

Ingredients:

- 2 apples, peeled and cored
- 2 teaspoons honey
- 1/2 teaspoon ground cinnamon

Instructions

1. Preheat oven to 350°F (175°C).

2. Place apples in a baking dish.

3. Drizzle with honey and sprinkle with cinnamon.

4. Bake for 20 minutes or until tender.

5. Serve warm.

Nutritional Values (per serving):

- Calories: 100 • Protein: 0g • Carbohydrates: 27g • Fat: 0g • Fiber: 4g

Soft Boiled Eggs

Servings: 2

Cooking Time: 10 minutes

Ingredients:

- 4 eggs

Instructions:

1. Bring a pot of water to a boil.

2. Carefully lower eggs into the boiling water.

3. Cook for 6 minutes for soft-boiled eggs.

4. Remove eggs and place in ice water for 1 minute.

5. Peel and serve.

Nutritional Values (per serving):

- Calories: 140 • Protein: 12g • Carbohydrates: 1g • Fat: 10g • Fiber: 0g

Mashed Banana on Toast

Servings: 2

Cooking Time: 5 minutes

Ingredients:

- 2 ripe bananas
- 2 slices white bread, toasted
- 1 tablespoon honey

Instructions

1. Mash bananas in a bowl.

2. Spread mashed banana on toasted bread.

3. Drizzle with honey.

4. Serve immediately.

Nutritional Values (per serving):

- Calories: 180 • Protein: 3g • Carbohydrates: 38g • Fat: 2g • Fiber: 3g

Egg Custard

Servings: 4

Cooking Time: 30 minutes

Ingredients:

- 2 cups skim milk
- 4 eggs
- 1/4 cup sugar
- 1 teaspoon vanilla extract
- Nutmeg (optional)

Instructions

1. Preheat oven to 325°F (160°C).
2. Heat milk in a saucepan until just warm.
3. In a bowl, whisk eggs, sugar, and vanilla extract.
4. Gradually add warm milk to egg mixture, stirring constantly.
5. Pour mixture into custard cups.
6. Place cups in a baking dish and fill with hot water halfway up the sides of the cups.
7. Bake for 25-30 minutes or until custard is set.
8. Sprinkle with nutmeg if desired and serve warm or chilled.

Nutritional Values (per serving):

• Calories: 130 • Protein: 6g • Carbohydrates: 15g • Fat: 5g • Fiber: 0g

Yogurt Parfait

Servings: 2

Cooking Time: 5 minutes

Ingredients

- 2 cups low-fat yogurt
- 1/2 cup canned fruit, drained and chopped
- 1 tablespoon honey

Instructions

1. Divide yogurt between two bowls.

2. Top with chopped fruit.

3. Drizzle with honey.

4. Serve immediately.

Nutritional Values (per serving):

- Calories: 140 • Protein: 6g • Carbohydrates: 28g • Fat: 2g • Fiber: 1g

Chapter 3: Lunch Recipes

Chicken and Rice Soup

Servings: 4

Cooking Time: 30 minutes

Ingredients

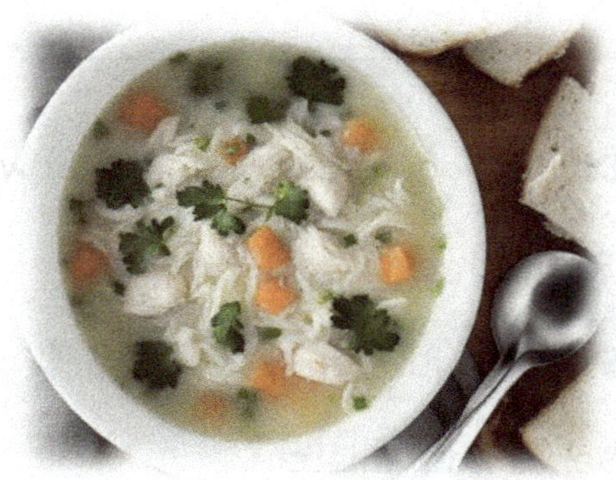

- 1 cup cooked chicken breast, shredded
- 1/2 cup white rice
- 4 cups low-sodium chicken broth
- 1 carrot, peeled and diced
- 1 celery stalk, diced
- 1/2 teaspoon salt
- 1/4 teaspoon pepper

Instructions

1. In a large pot, bring the chicken broth to a boil.

2. Add the rice, carrot, and celery.

3. Reduce heat and simmer for 20 minutes until rice and vegetables are tender.

4. Add shredded chicken, salt, and pepper.

5. Simmer for another 5 minutes.

6. Serve warm.

Nutritional Values (per serving):

• Calories: 180 • Protein: 15g • Carbohydrates: 22g • Fat: 3g • Fiber: 1g

Baked Fish with Mashed Potatoes

Servings: 4

Cooking Time: 30 minutes

Ingredients

- 4 white fish fillets (such as cod or haddock)
- 2 tablespoons olive oil
- 4 large potatoes, peeled and diced
- 1/2 cup skim milk
- 1 tablespoon butter
- 1/2 teaspoon salt
- 1/4 teaspoon pepper
- Lemon wedges (optional)

Instructions

1. Preheat oven to 375°F (190°C).

2. Place fish fillets on a baking sheet and drizzle with olive oil.

3. Bake for 15-20 minutes or until fish is cooked through.

4. Meanwhile, boil potatoes in a large pot until tender.

5. Drain and mash potatoes with milk, butter, salt, and pepper.

6. Serve fish with mashed potatoes and lemon wedges if desired.

Nutritional Values (per serving):

- Calories: 290 • Protein: 25g • Carbohydrates: 35g • Fat: 8g • Fiber: 3g

Creamy Tomato Soup

Servings: 4

Cooking Time: 25 minutes

Ingredients

- 4 cups canned tomatoes, pureed
- 2 cups low-sodium vegetable broth
- 1/2 cup skim milk
- 1 tablespoon olive oil
- 1 small onion, finely chopped
- 1 garlic clove, minced
- 1/2 teaspoon salt
- 1/4 teaspoon pepper

Instructions

1. Heat olive oil in a large pot over medium heat.

2. Add onion and garlic and cook until soft.

3. Stir in pureed tomatoes and vegetable broth.

4. Bring to a boil, then reduce heat and simmer for 15 minutes.

5. Stir in skim milk, salt, and pepper.

6. Serve warm.

Nutritional Values (per serving):

• Calories: 120 • Protein: 3g • Carbohydrates: 18g • Fat: 4g • Fiber: 4g

Turkey and Zucchini Meatballs

Servings: 4

Cooking Time: 30 minutes

Ingredients

- 1 pound ground turkey
- 1 small zucchini, grated
- 1 egg
- 1/4 cup breadcrumbs
- 1/2 teaspoon salt
- 1/4 teaspoon pepper
- 1 tablespoon olive oil
- 1 cup low-sodium marinara sauce

Instructions

1. Preheat oven to 375°F (190°C).
2. In a bowl, combine ground turkey, grated zucchini, egg, breadcrumbs, salt, and pepper.
3. Form mixture into meatballs.
4. Heat olive oil in a large skillet over medium heat.
5. Brown meatballs on all sides.
6. Transfer meatballs to a baking dish and cover with marinara sauce.
7. Bake for 20 minutes or until cooked through.
8. Serve warm.

Nutritional Values (per serving):

- Calories: 220 • Protein: 22g • Carbohydrates: 8g • Fat: 11g • Fiber: 1g

Chicken Salad Lettuce Wraps

Servings: 4

Cooking Time: 20 minutes

Ingredients

- 2 cups cooked chicken breast, shredded
- 1/4 cup low-fat mayonnaise
- 1/4 cup plain low-fat yogurt
- 1/2 teaspoon salt
- 1/4 teaspoon pepper
- 8 large lettuce leaves

Instructions

1. In a bowl, combine shredded chicken, mayonnaise, yogurt, salt, and pepper.

2. Spoon chicken salad onto lettuce leaves.

3. Roll up lettuce leaves and secure with toothpicks if needed.

4. Serve immediately.

Nutritional Values (per serving):

• Calories: 140 • Protein: 20g • Carbohydrates: 3g • Fat: 5g • Fiber: 1g

Creamy Spinach Soup

Servings: 4

Cooking Time: 30 minutes

Ingredients

- 4 cups fresh spinach, washed and chopped
- 1 small onion, chopped
- 1 garlic clove, minced
- 2 cups low-sodium chicken broth
- 1/2 cup skim milk
- 1 tablespoon olive oil
- 1/2 teaspoon salt
- 1/4 teaspoon pepper

Instructions

1. Heat olive oil in a large pot over medium heat.
2. Add onion and garlic and cook until soft.
3. Stir in spinach and cook until wilted.
4. Add chicken broth and bring to a boil.
5. Reduce heat and simmer for 15 minutes.
6. Puree soup using an immersion blender or in batches in a regular blender.
7. Stir in skim milk, salt, and pepper.
8. Serve warm.

Nutritional Values (per serving):

• Calories: 100 • Protein: 4g • Carbohydrates: 10g • Fat: 5g • Fiber: 2g

Turkey and Rice Casserole

Servings: 4

Cooking Time: 35 minutes

Ingredients

- 1 pound ground turkey
- 1 cup cooked white rice
- 1/2 cup low-fat sour cream
- 1/2 cup shredded low-fat cheese
- 1/2 teaspoon salt
- 1/4 teaspoon pepper
- 1 tablespoon olive oil

Instructions

1. Preheat oven to 350°F (175°C).

2. Heat olive oil in a skillet over medium heat.

3. Add ground turkey and cook until browned.

4. In a bowl, combine cooked turkey, rice, sour cream, cheese, salt, and pepper.

5. Transfer mixture to a baking dish.

6. Bake for 20 minutes or until heated through.

7. Serve warm.

Nutritional Values (per serving):

- Calories: 280 • Protein: 22g • Carbohydrates: 18g • Fat: 12g • Fiber: 1g

Creamy Chicken Pasta

Servings: 4

Cooking Time: 25 minutes

Ingredients

- 8 ounces pasta (such as penne or fusilli)
- 2 cups cooked chicken breast, shredded
- 1 cup skim milk
- 1/2 cup low-fat cream cheese
- 1/2 cup grated Parmesan cheese
- 1/2 teaspoon salt
- 1/4 teaspoon pepper

Instructions

1. Cook pasta according to package instructions.

2. In a saucepan, heat milk over medium heat.

3. Stir in cream cheese until melted and smooth.

4. Add shredded chicken, Parmesan cheese, salt, and pepper.

5. Cook until heated through.

6. Toss pasta with the creamy chicken sauce.

7. Serve warm.

Nutritional Values (per serving):

- Calories: 340 • Protein: 30g • Carbohydrates: 30g • Fat: 10g • Fiber: 2g

Baked Chicken and Vegetables

Servings: 4

Cooking Time: 40 minutes

Ingredients

- 4 chicken breasts
- 2 carrots, peeled and sliced
- 2 zucchini, sliced
- 2 tablespoons olive oil
- 1 teaspoon salt
- 1/2 teaspoon pepper
- 1 teaspoon dried thyme

Instructions

1. Preheat oven to 375°F (190°C).
2. Place chicken breasts and vegetables on a baking sheet.
3. Drizzle with olive oil and season with salt, pepper, and thyme.
4. Bake for 30-35 minutes or until chicken is cooked through and vegetables are tender.
5. Serve warm.

Nutritional Values (per serving):

• Calories: 260 • Protein: 30g • Carbohydrates: 10g • Fat: 10g • Fiber: 3g

Tuna Salad

Servings: 2

Cooking Time: 10 minutes

Ingredients

- 1 can tuna in water, drained
- 1/4 cup low-fat mayonnaise
- 1 tablespoon lemon juice
- 1/4 teaspoon salt
- 1/4 teaspoon pepper
- 2 cups mixed greens

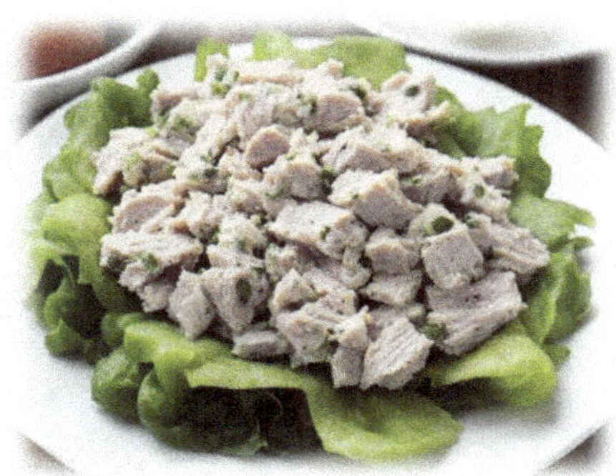

Instructions

1. In a bowl, combine tuna, mayonnaise, lemon juice, salt, and pepper.

2. Serve tuna salad over mixed greens.

3. Serve immediately.

Nutritional Values (per serving):

- Calories: 180 • Protein: 22g • Carbohydrates: 2g • Fat: 9g • Fiber: 1g

Vegetable Stir-Fry

Servings: 4

Cooking Time: 20 minutes

Ingredients

- 1 cup broccoli florets
- 1 red bell pepper, sliced
- 1 carrot, peeled and sliced
- 1 zucchini, sliced
- 1 tablespoon olive oil
- 2 tablespoons low-sodium soy sauce
- 1/2 teaspoon ground ginger

Instructions

1. Heat olive oil in a large skillet over medium heat.

2. Add broccoli, bell pepper, carrot, and zucchini.

3. Stir-fry for 5-7 minutes until vegetables are tender-crisp.

4. Stir in soy sauce and ginger.

5. Cook for another 2 minutes.

6. Serve warm.

Nutritional Values (per serving):

• Calories: 90 • Protein: 2g • Carbohydrates: 12g • Fat: 4g • Fiber: 3g

Potato and Leek Soup

Servings: 4

Cooking Time: 30 minutes

Ingredients

- 4 large potatoes, peeled and diced
- 2 leeks, washed and sliced
- 4 cups low-sodium vegetable broth
- 1/2 cup skim milk
- 1 tablespoon olive oil
- 1/2 teaspoon salt
- 1/4 teaspoon pepper

Instructions

1. Heat olive oil in a large pot over medium heat.

2. Add leeks and cook until soft.

3. Stir in potatoes and vegetable broth.

4. Bring to a boil, then reduce heat and simmer for 20 minutes.

5. Puree soup using an immersion blender or in batches in a regular blender.

6. Stir in skim milk, salt, and pepper.

7. Serve warm.

Nutritional Values (per serving):

- Calories: 160 • Protein: 4g • Carbohydrates: 32g • Fat: 2g • Fiber: 3g

Shrimp and Quinoa Salad

Servings: 4

Cooking Time: 25 minutes

Ingredients

- 1 cup quinoa
- 2 cups water
- 1 pound cooked shrimp, peeled and deveined
- 1/2 cup cherry tomatoes, halved
- 1/4 cup chopped fresh parsley
- 1/4 cup lemon juice
- 2 tablespoons olive oil
- 1/2 teaspoon salt
- 1/4 teaspoon pepper

Instructions

1. Rinse quinoa under cold water.

2. In a saucepan, bring water to a boil.

3. Add quinoa, reduce heat, cover, and simmer for 15 minutes.

4. Fluff quinoa with a fork and let cool.

5. In a large bowl, combine quinoa, shrimp, cherry tomatoes, and parsley.

6. In a small bowl, whisk together lemon juice, olive oil, salt, and pepper.

7. Pour dressing over salad and toss to combine.

8. Serve chilled.

Nutritional Values (per serving):

- Calories: 250 • Protein: 20g • Carbohydrates: 26g • Fat: 8g • Fiber: 3g

Chicken and Vegetable Skewers

Servings: 4

Cooking Time: 30 minutes

Ingredients

- 4 chicken breasts, cut into cubes
- 1 red bell pepper, cut into squares
- 1 zucchini, sliced
- 1 red onion, cut into squares
- 2 tablespoons olive oil
- 1 teaspoon dried oregano
- 1/2 teaspoon salt
- 1/4 teaspoon pepper

Instructions

1. Preheat grill to medium-high heat.
2. Thread chicken, bell pepper, zucchini, and onion onto skewers.
3. Brush with olive oil and season with oregano, salt, and pepper.
4. Grill for 10-15 minutes, turning occasionally, until chicken is cooked through and vegetables are tender.
5. Serve warm.

Nutritional Values (per serving):

- Calories: 240 • Protein: 26g • Carbohydrates: 8g • Fat: 12g • Fiber: 2g

Turkey and Sweet Potato Patties

Servings: 4

Cooking Time: 25 minutes

Ingredients

- 1 pound ground turkey
- 1 cup mashed sweet potatoes
- 1 egg
- 1/4 cup breadcrumbs
- 1/2 teaspoon salt
- 1/4 teaspoon pepper
- 1 tablespoon olive oil

Instructions

1. In a large bowl, combine ground turkey, mashed sweet potatoes, egg, breadcrumbs, salt, and pepper.
2. Form mixture into patties.
3. Heat olive oil in a large skillet over medium heat.
4. Cook patties for 5-7 minutes on each side or until golden brown and cooked through.
5. Serve warm.

Nutritional Values (per serving):

• Calories: 210 • Protein: 18g • Carbohydrates: 12g • Fat: 10g • Fiber: 2g

Chapter 4: Dinner Recipes

Lemon Herb Salmon

Servings: 4

Cooking Time: 25 minutes

Ingredients

- 4 salmon fillets
- 2 tablespoons olive oil
- 1 lemon, sliced
- 1 teaspoon dried oregano
- 1 teaspoon dried thyme
- 1/2 teaspoon salt
- 1/4 teaspoon pepper

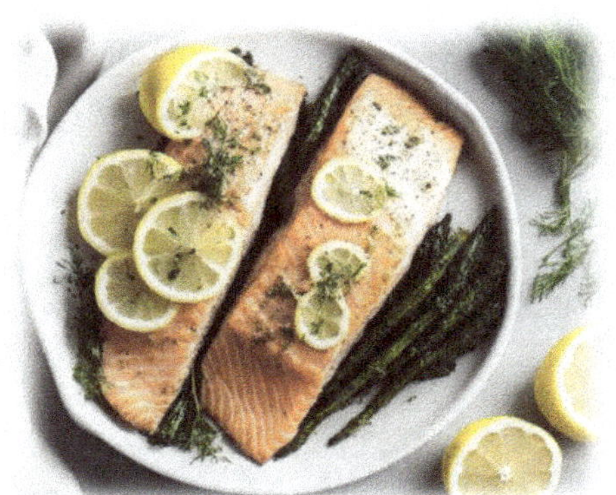

Instructions

1. Preheat oven to 375°F (190°C).
2. Place salmon fillets on a baking sheet.
3. Drizzle with olive oil and season with oregano, thyme, salt, and pepper.
4. Top each fillet with lemon slices.
5. Bake for 20 minutes or until salmon is cooked through and flakes easily with a fork.
6. Serve warm.

Nutritional Values (per serving):

- Calories: 280 • Protein: 25g • Carbohydrates: 2g • Fat: 18g • Fiber: 1g

Turkey Meatballs with Zucchini Noodles

Servings: 4

Cooking Time: 30 minutes

Ingredients

- 1 pound ground turkey
- 1/4 cup breadcrumbs
- 1 egg
- 1/4 cup grated Parmesan cheese
- 1 teaspoon dried basil
- 1 teaspoon dried oregano
- 1/2 teaspoon salt
- 1/4 teaspoon pepper
- 4 zucchinis, spiralized
- 2 tablespoons olive oil

Instructions

1. Preheat oven to 400°F (200°C).
2. In a large bowl, combine ground turkey, breadcrumbs, egg, Parmesan cheese, basil, oregano, salt, and pepper.
3. Form mixture into meatballs and place on a baking sheet.
4. Bake for 20 minutes or until meatballs are cooked through.
5. While meatballs are baking, heat olive oil in a large skillet over medium heat.
6. Add spiralized zucchini and cook for 5-7 minutes until tender.
7. Serve meatballs over zucchini noodles.

Nutritional Values (per serving):

• Calories: 280 • Protein: 26g • Carbohydrates: 10g • Fat: 16g • Fiber: 3g

Quinoa Stuffed Bell Peppers

Servings: 4

Cooking Time: 45 minutes

Ingredients

- 4 bell peppers, tops removed and seeds removed
- 1 cup cooked quinoa
- 1 cup black beans, rinsed and drained
- 1 cup corn kernels
- 1 cup diced tomatoes
- 1 teaspoon cumin
- 1/2 teaspoon salt
- 1/4 teaspoon pepper
- 1/2 cup shredded cheddar cheese

Instructions

1. Preheat oven to 375°F (190°C).
2. In a large bowl, combine cooked quinoa, black beans, corn, tomatoes, cumin, salt, and pepper.
3. Stuff each bell pepper with the quinoa mixture and place in a baking dish.
4. Cover with foil and bake for 30 minutes.
5. Remove foil, sprinkle with cheddar cheese, and bake for an additional 10 minutes.
6. Serve warm.

Nutritional Values (per serving):

- Calories: 300 • Protein: 14g • Carbohydrates: 46g • Fat: 9g • Fiber: 9g

Chicken and Broccoli Stir-Fry

Servings: 4

Cooking Time: 20 minutes

Ingredients

- 1 pound chicken breast, sliced into strips
- 2 cups broccoli florets
- 1 red bell pepper, sliced
- 1 tablespoon olive oil
- 2 tablespoons low-sodium soy sauce
- 1 tablespoon honey
- 1 teaspoon grated ginger
- 1 garlic clove, minced

Instructions

1. Heat olive oil in a large skillet over medium-high heat.
2. Add chicken strips and cook until browned and cooked through.
3. Remove chicken from skillet and set aside.
4. In the same skillet, add broccoli and bell pepper. Cook for 5-7 minutes until tender.
5. In a small bowl, mix soy sauce, honey, ginger, and garlic.
6. Return chicken to the skillet and pour sauce over the top.
7. Cook for another 2-3 minutes until everything is heated through.
8. Serve warm.

Nutritional Values (per serving):

• Calories: 280 • Protein: 28g • Carbohydrates: 18g • Fat: 10g • Fiber: 4g

Baked Cod with Vegetables

Servings: 4

Cooking Time: 35 minutes

Ingredients

- 4 cod fillets
- 1 cup cherry tomatoes, halved
- 1 zucchini, sliced
- 1 red onion, sliced
- 2 tablespoons olive oil
- 1 lemon, juiced
- 1 teaspoon dried oregano
- 1/2 teaspoon salt
- 1/4 teaspoon pepper

Instructions

1. Preheat oven to 375°F (190°C).
2. Place cod fillets and vegetables on a baking sheet.
3. Drizzle with olive oil and lemon juice, and season with oregano, salt, and pepper.
4. Bake for 25-30 minutes or until cod is cooked through and vegetables are tender.
5. Serve warm.

Nutritional Values (per serving):

• Calories: 250 • Protein: 25g • Carbohydrates: 10g • Fat: 12g • Fiber: 3g

Beef and Vegetable Kebabs

Servings: 4

Cooking Time: 30 minutes

Ingredients

- 1-pound beef sirloin, cut into cubes
- 1 red bell pepper, cut into squares
- 1 yellow bell pepper, cut into squares
- 1 zucchini, sliced
- 1 red onion, cut into squares
- 2 tablespoons olive oil
- 1 teaspoon dried rosemary
- 1/2 teaspoon salt
- 1/4 teaspoon pepper

Instructions

1. Preheat grill to medium-high heat.
2. Thread beef and vegetables onto skewers.
3. Brush with olive oil and season with rosemary, salt, and pepper.
4. Grill for 10-15 minutes, turning occasionally, until beef is cooked to desired doneness and vegetables are tender.
5. Serve warm.

Nutritional Values (per serving):

• Calories: 320 • Protein: 28g • Carbohydrates: 10g • Fat: 18g • Fiber: 3g

Spaghetti Squash with Tomato Sauce

Servings: 4

Cooking Time: 45 minutes

Ingredients

- 1 large spaghetti squash
- 2 cups tomato sauce
- 1/2 cup grated Parmesan cheese
- 1 tablespoon olive oil
- 1 teaspoon dried basil
- 1/2 teaspoon salt
- 1/4 teaspoon pepper

Instructions

1. Preheat oven to 375°F (190°C).
2. Cut spaghetti squash in half lengthwise and scoop out seeds.
3. Place squash halves cut-side down on a baking sheet and bake for 35-40 minutes until tender.
4. Using a fork, scrape the squash to create spaghetti-like strands.
5. In a large skillet, heat olive oil over medium heat.
6. Add tomato sauce, basil, salt, and pepper. Cook for 5 minutes until heated through.
7. Add spaghetti squash strands to the skillet and toss to combine.
8. Serve topped with Parmesan cheese.

Nutritional Values (per serving):

• Calories: 210 • Protein: 7g • Carbohydrates: 30g • Fat: 9g • Fiber: 5g

Baked Chicken with Sweet Potatoes

Servings: 4

Cooking Time: 45 minutes

Ingredients

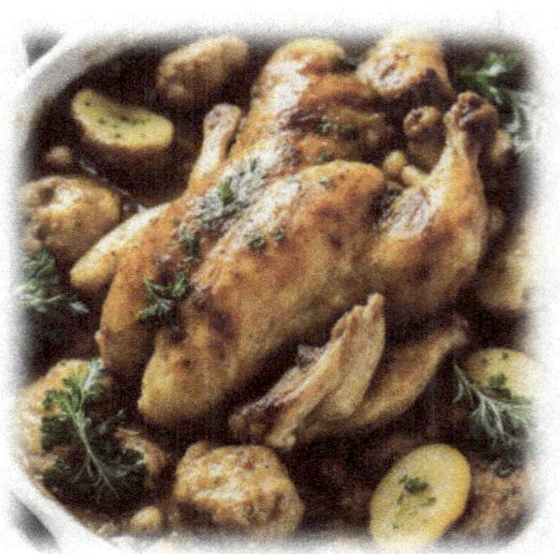

- 4 chicken breasts
- 2 large sweet potatoes, peeled and diced
- 2 tablespoons olive oil
- 1 teaspoon paprika
- 1/2 teaspoon garlic powder
- 1/2 teaspoon salt
- 1/4 teaspoon pepper

Instructions

1. Preheat oven to 400°F (200°C).
2. Place chicken breasts and sweet potatoes on a baking sheet.
3. Drizzle with olive oil and season with paprika, garlic powder, salt, and pepper.
4. Bake for 35-40 minutes until chicken is cooked through and sweet potatoes are tender.
5. Serve warm.

Nutritional Values (per serving):

- Calories: 350 • Protein: 30g • Carbohydrates: 28g • Fat: 12g • Fiber: 5g

Shrimp and Asparagus Stir-Fry

Servings: 4

Cooking Time: 20 minutes

Ingredients

- 1 pound shrimp, peeled and deveined
- 1 bunch asparagus, trimmed and cut into pieces
- 1 red bell pepper, sliced
- 2 tablespoons olive oil
- 2 tablespoons low-sodium soy sauce
- 1 tablespoon lemon juice
- 1 garlic clove, minced

Instructions

1. Heat olive oil in a large skillet over medium-high heat.
2. Add shrimp and cook until pink and opaque, about 2-3 minutes per side.
3. Remove shrimp from skillet and set aside.
4. In the same skillet, add asparagus and bell pepper. Cook for 5-7 minutes until tender.
5. Return shrimp to the skillet and add soy sauce, lemon juice, and garlic.
6. Cook for another 2-3 minutes until everything is heated through.
7. Serve warm.

Nutritional Values (per serving):

- Calories: 230 • Protein: 25g • Carbohydrates: 8g • Fat: 12g • Fiber: 3g

Turkey and Spinach Stuffed Peppers

Servings: 4

Cooking Time: 45 minutes

Ingredients

- 4 bell peppers, tops removed and seeds removed
- 1 pound ground turkey
- 1 cup cooked quinoa
- 1 cup fresh spinach, chopped
- 1 small onion, diced
- 1 garlic clove, minced
- 1/2 teaspoon salt
- 1/4 teaspoon pepper
- 1/2 cup shredded mozzarella cheese

Instructions

1. Preheat oven to 375°F (190°C).
2. In a large skillet, cook ground turkey over medium heat until browned and cooked through.
3. Add onion and garlic to the skillet and cook until soft.
4. Stir in cooked quinoa, spinach, salt, and pepper.
5. Stuff each bell pepper with the turkey mixture and place in a baking dish.
6. Cover with foil and bake for 30 minutes.
7. Remove foil, sprinkle with mozzarella cheese, and bake for an additional 10 minutes.
8. Serve warm.

Nutritional Values (per serving):

• Calories: 320 • Protein: 28g • Carbohydrates: 25g • Fat: 12g • Fiber: 5g

Lentil and Vegetable Stew

Servings: 4

Cooking Time: 40 minutes

Ingredients

- 1 cup green lentils
- 4 cups low-sodium vegetable broth
- 1 carrot, diced
- 1 celery stalk, diced
- 1 small onion, chopped
- 1 garlic clove, minced
- 1 tablespoon olive oil
- 1 teaspoon dried thyme
- 1/2 teaspoon salt
- 1/4 teaspoon pepper

Instructions

1. Heat olive oil in a large pot over medium heat.
2. Add onion, carrot, celery, and garlic. Cook until vegetables are soft.
3. Stir in lentils, vegetable broth, thyme, salt, and pepper.
4. Bring to a boil, then reduce heat and simmer for 30-35 minutes until lentils are tender.
5. Serve warm.

Nutritional Values (per serving):

- Calories: 220 • Protein: 12g • Carbohydrates: 36g • Fat: 4g • Fiber: 15g

Chicken and Rice Casserole

Servings: 4

Cooking Time: 50 minutes

Ingredients

- 2 cups cooked brown rice
- 1-pound chicken breast, diced
- 1 cup broccoli florets
- 1 cup low-fat milk
- 1/2 cup shredded cheddar cheese
- 1/4 cup breadcrumbs
- 1 tablespoon olive oil
- 1/2 teaspoon salt
- 1/4 teaspoon pepper

Instructions

1. Preheat oven to 375°F (190°C).
2. In a large skillet, heat olive oil over medium heat.
3. Add diced chicken and cook until browned and cooked through.
4. In a large bowl, combine cooked rice, chicken, broccoli, milk, salt, and pepper.
5. Transfer mixture to a baking dish and top with cheddar cheese and breadcrumbs.
6. Bake for 25-30 minutes until cheese is melted and casserole is heated through.
7. Serve warm.

Nutritional Values (per serving):

• Calories: 380 • Protein: 30g • Carbohydrates: 40g • Fat: 12g • Fiber: 4g

Baked Eggplant Parmesan

Servings: 4

Cooking Time: 50 minutes

Ingredients

- 1 large eggplant, sliced
- 1 cup breadcrumbs
- 1/2 cup grated Parmesan cheese
- 2 eggs, beaten
- 2 cups marinara sauce
- 1 cup shredded mozzarella cheese
- 1 tablespoon olive oil
- 1/2 teaspoon salt
- 1/4 teaspoon pepper

Instructions

1. Preheat oven to 375°F (190°C).
2. In a shallow dish, mix breadcrumbs and Parmesan cheese.
3. Dip eggplant slices into beaten eggs, then coat with breadcrumb mixture.
4. Place coated eggplant slices on a baking sheet and drizzle with olive oil.
5. Bake for 20 minutes, turning once, until golden brown.
6. In a baking dish, spread a thin layer of marinara sauce.
7. Layer baked eggplant slices over the sauce, then top with more sauce and mozzarella cheese.
8. Repeat layers until all ingredients are used, ending with cheese on top.
9. Bake for an additional 20-25 minutes until cheese is melted and bubbly.
10. Serve warm.

Nutritional Values (per serving):

• Calories: 340 • Protein: 18g • Carbohydrates: 40g • Fat: 14g • Fiber: 8g

Stuffed Portobello Mushrooms

Servings: 4

Cooking Time: 30 minutes

Ingredients

- 4 large Portobello mushrooms, stems removed
- 1 cup cooked quinoa
- 1/2 cup diced tomatoes
- 1/4 cup crumbled feta cheese
- 1 small onion, chopped
- 1 garlic clove, minced
- 1 tablespoon olive oil
- 1/2 teaspoon dried oregano
- 1/2 teaspoon salt
- 1/4 teaspoon pepper

Instructions

1. Preheat oven to 375°F (190°C).
2. In a large skillet, heat olive oil over medium heat.
3. Add onion and garlic and cook until soft.
4. Stir in cooked quinoa, tomatoes, feta cheese, oregano, salt, and pepper.
5. Stuff each Portobello mushroom with the quinoa mixture and place on a baking sheet.
6. Bake for 20-25 minutes until mushrooms are tender.
7. Serve warm.

Nutritional Values (per serving):

• Calories: 220 • Protein: 9g • Carbohydrates: 24g • Fat: 10g • Fiber: 5g

Honey Mustard Glazed Chicken

Servings: 4

Cooking Time: 30 minutes

Ingredients

- 4 chicken breasts
- 1/4 cup honey
- 2 tablespoons Dijon mustard
- 1 tablespoon olive oil
- 1 garlic clove, minced
- 1/2 teaspoon salt
- 1/4 teaspoon pepper

Instructions

1. Preheat oven to 375°F (190°C).

2. In a small bowl, mix honey, Dijon mustard, olive oil, garlic, salt, and pepper.

3. Place chicken breasts in a baking dish and brush with honey mustard mixture.

4. Bake for 25-30 minutes until chicken is cooked through.

5. Serve warm.

Nutritional Values (per serving):

- Calories: 320 • Protein: 28g • Carbohydrates: 18g • Fat: 14g • Fiber: 0g

Chapter 5: Snacks and Small Bites

Greek Yogurt Parfait

Servings: 4

Cooking Time: 10 minutes

Ingredients

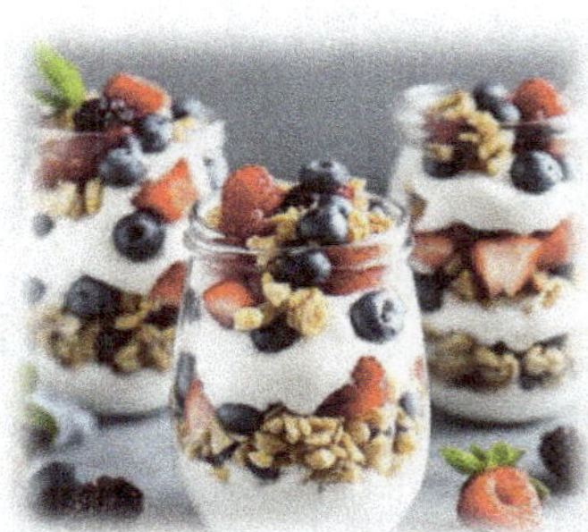

- 2 cups Greek yogurt
- 1 cup mixed berries (blueberries, strawberries, raspberries)
- 1/2 cup granola
- 2 tablespoons honey

Instructions

1. In four glasses, layer Greek yogurt, mixed berries, and granola.

2. Drizzle honey over the top.

3. Serve immediately.

Nutritional Values (per serving):

- Calories: 180 • Protein: 10g • Carbohydrates: 28g • Fat: 4g • Fiber: 3g

Baked Zucchini Chips

Servings: 4

Cooking Time: 30 minutes

Ingredients

- 2 large zucchinis, thinly sliced
- 2 tablespoons olive oil
- 1/2 teaspoon salt
- 1/4 teaspoon pepper
- 1/2 teaspoon garlic powder

Instructions

1. Preheat oven to 225°F (110°C).
2. Place zucchini slices in a bowl and toss with olive oil, salt, pepper, and garlic powder.
3. Arrange slices on a baking sheet in a single layer.
4. Bake for 2 hours or until crispy, flipping halfway through.
5. Serve immediately.

Nutritional Values (per serving):

- Calories: 70 • Protein: 1g • Carbohydrates: 5g • Fat: 5g • Fiber: 1g

Apple Slices with Almond Butter

Servings: 4

Cooking Time: 10 minutes

Ingredients

- 2 large apples, sliced
- 1/2 cup almond butter

Instructions

1. Arrange apple slices on a plate.

2. Serve with almond butter on the side for dipping.

Nutritional Values (per serving):

• Calories: 160 • Protein: 4g • Carbohydrates: 20g • Fat: 8g • Fiber: 4g

Hummus and Veggie Sticks

Servings: 4

Cooking Time: 15 minutes

Ingredients

- 2 cups hummus
- 2 carrots, cut into sticks
- 2 celery stalks, cut into sticks
- 1 cucumber, cut into sticks

Instructions

1. Place hummus in a bowl.

2. Arrange veggie sticks around the bowl.

3. Serve immediately.

Nutritional Values (per serving):

• Calories: 150 • Protein: 4g • Carbohydrates: 18g • Fat: 8g • Fiber: 6g

Deviled Eggs

Servings: 4

Cooking Time: 20 minutes

Ingredients

- 6 large eggs
- 2 tablespoons mayonnaise
- 1 teaspoon Dijon mustard
- 1/4 teaspoon paprika
- 1/4 teaspoon salt
- 1/4 teaspoon pepper

Instructions

1. Place eggs in a pot and cover with water. Bring to a boil and cook for 10 minutes.
2. Remove eggs, cool under running water, and peel.
3. Slice eggs in half lengthwise and remove yolks.
4. In a bowl, mash yolks with mayonnaise, mustard, salt, and pepper.
5. Spoon yolk mixture back into egg whites and sprinkle with paprika.
6. Serve immediately.

Nutritional Values (per serving):

- Calories: 120 • Protein: 6g • Carbohydrates: 1g • Fat: 10g • Fiber: 0g

Cottage Cheese with Pineapple

Servings: 4

Cooking Time: 10 minutes

Ingredients

- 2 cups cottage cheese
- 1 cup pineapple chunks (fresh or canned)

Instructions

1. In four bowls, divide cottage cheese.

2. Top with pineapple chunks.

3. Serve immediately.

Nutritional Values (per serving):

- Calories: 120 • Protein: 12g • Carbohydrates: 15g • Fat: 3g • Fiber: 1g

Smoothie Pops

Servings: 4

Cooking Time: 10 minutes (plus freezing time)

Ingredients

- 1 cup Greek yogurt
- 1 cup mixed berries (blueberries, strawberries, raspberries)
- 1 banana
- 1/2 cup orange juice

Instructions

1. In a blender, combine Greek yogurt, mixed berries, banana, and orange juice. Blend until smooth.
2. Pour mixture into popsicle molds.
3. Freeze for at least 4 hours or until solid.
4. Serve frozen.

Nutritional Values (per serving):

- Calories: 100 • Protein: 4g • Carbohydrates: 20g • Fat: 1g • Fiber: 3g

Caprese Skewers

Servings: 4

Cooking Time: 15 minutes

Ingredients

- 1 cup cherry tomatoes
- 1 cup fresh mozzarella balls
- 1/4 cup fresh basil leaves
- 2 tablespoons balsamic glaze

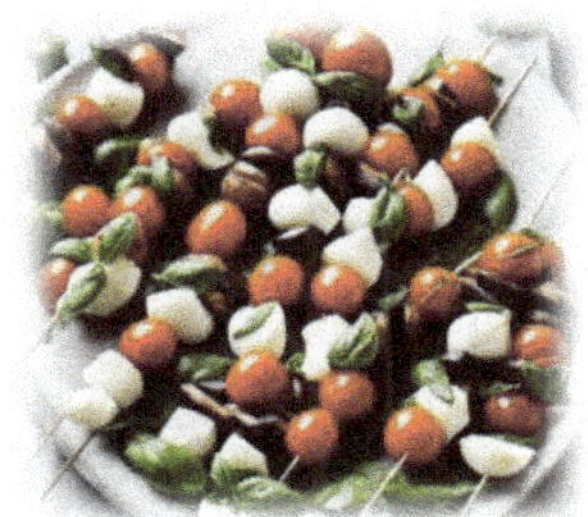

Instructions

1. Thread cherry tomatoes, mozzarella balls, and basil leaves onto skewers.

2. Drizzle with balsamic glaze.

3. Serve immediately.

Nutritional Values (per serving):

- Calories: 130 • Protein: 7g • Carbohydrates: 8g • Fat: 8g • Fiber: 1g

Rice Cakes with Avocado

Servings: 4

Cooking Time: 10 minutes

Ingredients

- 4 rice cakes
- 2 avocados, mashed
- 1/4 teaspoon salt
- 1/4 teaspoon pepper

Instructions

1. Spread mashed avocado on rice cakes.

2. Season with salt and pepper.

3. Serve immediately.

Nutritional Values (per serving):

• Calories: 160 • Protein: 3g • Carbohydrates: 22g • Fat: 8g • Fiber: 5g

Trail Mix

Servings: 4

Cooking Time: 5 minutes

Ingredients

- 1/2 cup almonds
- 1/2 cup cashews
- 1/2 cup dried cranberries
- 1/2 cup dark chocolate chips

Instructions

1. In a large bowl, combine almonds, cashews, dried cranberries, and dark chocolate chips.
2. Mix well.
3. Serve immediately or store in an airtight container.

Nutritional Values (per serving):

• Calories: 220 • Protein: 6g • Carbohydrates: 26g • Fat: 12g • Fiber: 3g

Cucumber Bites with Cream Cheese

Servings: 4

Cooking Time: 10 minutes

Ingredients

- 1 large cucumber, sliced
- 1/2 cup cream cheese
- 1 tablespoon fresh dill, chopped
- 1/4 teaspoon salt
- 1/4 teaspoon pepper

Instructions

1. In a bowl, mix cream cheese, dill, salt, and pepper.

2. Spread mixture onto cucumber slices.

3. Serve immediately.

Nutritional Values (per serving):

- Calories: 90 • Protein: 2g • Carbohydrates: 4g • Fat: 8g • Fiber: 1g

Banana Oat Energy Bites

Servings: 4

Cooking Time: 15 minutes

Ingredients

- 1 cup rolled oats
- 1/2 cup peanut butter
- 1/4 cup honey
- 1 banana, mashed

Instructions

1. In a large bowl, combine rolled oats, peanut butter, honey, and mashed banana. Mix well.
2. Roll mixture into small balls.
3. Chill in the refrigerator for at least 30 minutes.
4. Serve chilled.

Nutritional Values (per serving):

- Calories: 180 • Protein: 5g • Carbohydrates: 27g • Fat: 7g • Fiber: 3g

Baked Sweet Potato Fries

Servings: 4

Cooking Time: 30 minutes

Ingredients

- 2 large sweet potatoes, peeled and cut into fries
- 2 tablespoons olive oil
- 1/2 teaspoon salt
- 1/4 teaspoon pepper
- 1/2 teaspoon paprika

Instructions

1. Preheat oven to 425°F (220°C).

2. In a large bowl, toss sweet potato fries with olive oil, salt, pepper, and paprika.

3. Arrange fries on a baking sheet in a single layer.

4. Bake for 25-30 minutes, flipping halfway through, until crispy.

5. Serve immediately.

Nutritional Values (per serving):

• Calories: 150 • Protein: 2g • Carbohydrates: 25g • Fat: 5g • Fiber: 4g

Mini Quiche Cups

Servings: 4

Cooking Time: 25 minutes

Ingredients

- 4 eggs
- 1/2 cup milk
- 1/2 cup shredded cheddar cheese
- 1/4 cup diced ham
- 1/4 cup chopped spinach
- 1/4 teaspoon salt
- 1/4 teaspoon pepper

Instructions

1. Preheat oven to 375°F (190°C).

2. In a bowl, whisk together eggs, milk, cheese, ham, spinach, salt, and pepper.

3. Pour mixture into a greased mini muffin tin.

4. Bake for 20-25 minutes until quiches are set and golden brown.

5. Serve warm.

Nutritional Values (per serving):

• Calories: 120 • Protein: 8g • Carbohydrates: 2g • Fat: 8g • Fiber: 0g

Mango Salsa

Servings: 4

Cooking Time: 15 minutes

Ingredients

- 2 ripe mangoes, diced
- 1 red bell pepper, diced
- 1/2 red onion, diced
- 1/4 cup fresh cilantro, chopped
- 1 lime, juiced
- 1/4 teaspoon salt
- 1/4 teaspoon pepper

Instructions

1. In a large bowl, combine mangoes, bell pepper, red onion, and cilantro.

2. Add lime juice, salt, and pepper. Mix well.

3. Serve immediately with tortilla chips or as a topping for grilled meats.

Nutritional Values (per serving):

- Calories: 90 • Protein: 1g • Carbohydrates: 22g • Fat: 0g • Fiber: 3g

Vanilla Pudding

Servings: 4

Cooking Time: 20 minutes

Ingredients

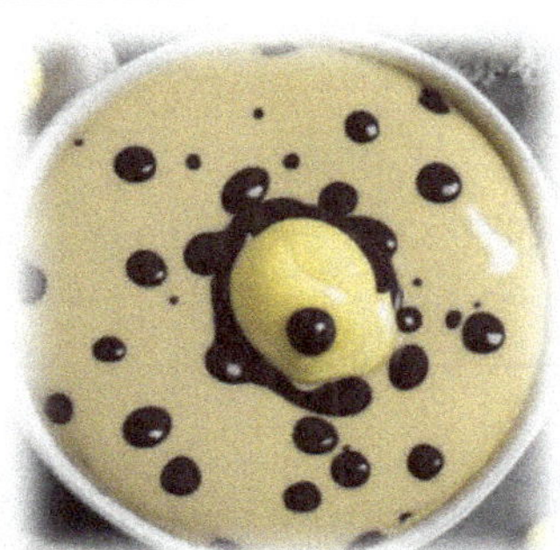

- 2 cups milk
- 1/2 cup sugar
- 3 tablespoons cornstarch
- 1/4 teaspoon salt
- 1 teaspoon vanilla extract

Instructions

1. In a medium saucepan, combine milk, sugar, cornstarch, and salt. Whisk until smooth.
2. Cook over medium heat, stirring constantly, until mixture thickens and comes to a boil.
3. Remove from heat and stir in vanilla extract.
4. Pour into serving dishes and chill in the refrigerator for at least 2 hours before serving.

Nutritional Values (per serving):

- Calories: 150 • Protein: 3g • Carbohydrates: 30g • Fat: 3g • Fiber: 0g

Chocolate Avocado Mousse

Servings: 4

Cooking Time: 15 minutes

Ingredients

- 2 ripe avocados
- 1/4 cup cocoa powder
- 1/4 cup honey
- 1/4 cup almond milk
- 1 teaspoon vanilla extract

Instructions

1. In a blender, combine avocados, cocoa powder, honey, almond milk, and vanilla extract. Blend until smooth.
2. Spoon mixture into serving dishes.
3. Chill in the refrigerator for at least 30 minutes before serving.

Nutritional Values (per serving):

• Calories: 200 • Protein: 3g • Carbohydrates: 30g • Fat: 12g • Fiber: 7g

Chia Seed Pudding

Servings: 4

Cooking Time: 10 minutes (plus chilling time)

Ingredients

- 2 cups almond milk
- 1/2 cup chia seeds
- 1/4 cup maple syrup
- 1 teaspoon vanilla extract

Instructions

1. In a large bowl, whisk together almond milk, chia seeds, maple syrup, and vanilla extract.
2. Cover and chill in the refrigerator for at least 4 hours or overnight.
3. Stir well before serving.

Nutritional Values (per serving):

• Calories: 200 • Protein: 5g • Carbohydrates: 25g • Fat: 10g • Fiber: 10g

Berry Compote

Servings: 4

Cooking Time: 15 minutes

Ingredients

- 2 cups mixed berries (strawberries, blueberries, raspberries)
- 1/4 cup sugar
- 1 tablespoon lemon juice

Instructions

1. In a medium saucepan, combine berries, sugar, and lemon juice. Cook over medium heat, stirring occasionally, until berries are soft and mixture is thickened, about 10-15 minutes.
2. Serve warm or chilled.

Nutritional Values (per serving):

• Calories: 80 • Protein: 1g • Carbohydrates: 20g • Fat: 0g • Fiber: 4g

Coconut Macaroons

Servings: 4

Cooking Time: 25 minutes

Ingredients

- 2 cups shredded coconut
- 1/2 cup sweetened condensed milk
- 1 teaspoon vanilla extract

Instructions

1. Preheat oven to 325°F (165°C).
2. In a large bowl, combine shredded coconut, sweetened condensed milk, and vanilla extract. Mix well.
3. Drop by tablespoonfuls onto a greased baking sheet.
4. Bake for 20-25 minutes, until golden brown.
5. Serve warm or at room temperature.

Nutritional Values (per serving):

- Calories: 220 • Protein: 2g • Carbohydrates: 30g • Fat: 10g • Fiber: 3g

Rice Pudding

Servings: 4

Cooking Time: 30 minutes

Ingredients

- 1/2 cup rice
- 2 cups milk
- 1/4 cup sugar
- 1 teaspoon vanilla extract
- 1/4 teaspoon cinnamon

Instructions

1. In a medium saucepan, combine rice, milk, and sugar. Cook over medium heat, stirring frequently, until rice is tender and mixture is thickened, about 25-30 minutes.
2. Remove from heat and stir in vanilla extract and cinnamon.
3. Serve warm or chilled.

Nutritional Values (per serving):

• Calories: 150 • Protein: 4g • Carbohydrates: 30g • Fat: 2g • Fiber: 1g

Lemon Sorbet

Servings: 4

Cooking Time: 15 minutes (plus freezing time)

Ingredients

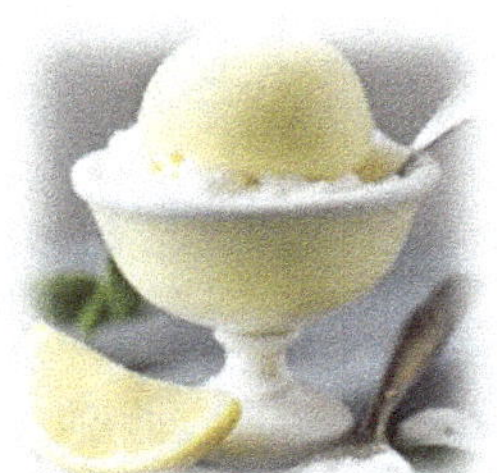

- 1 cup water
- 1 cup sugar
- 1 cup fresh lemon juice
- 1 tablespoon lemon zest

Instructions

1. In a small saucepan, combine water and sugar. Cook over medium heat, stirring constantly, until sugar is dissolved.
2. Remove from heat and stir in lemon juice and zest.
3. Pour mixture into a shallow dish and freeze for 4-6 hours, stirring every hour.
4. Serve frozen.

Nutritional Values (per serving):

- Calories: 150 • Protein: 0g • Carbohydrates: 39g • Fat: 0g • Fiber: 0g

Peach Sorbet

Servings: 4

Cooking Time: 15 minutes (plus freezing time)

Ingredients

- 4 ripe peaches, peeled and sliced
- 1/4 cup sugar
- 1 tablespoon lemon juice

Instructions

1. In a blender, combine peaches, sugar, and lemon juice. Blend until smooth.

2. Pour mixture into a shallow dish and freeze for 4-6 hours, stirring every hour.

3. Serve frozen.

Nutritional Values (per serving):

• Calories: 100 • Protein: 1g • Carbohydrates: 26g • Fat: 0g • Fiber: 2g

Banana Ice Cream

Servings: 4

Cooking Time: 10 minutes (plus freezing time)

Ingredients

- 4 ripe bananas, sliced and frozen
- 1/4 cup almond milk
- 1 teaspoon vanilla extract

Instructions

1. In a blender, combine frozen bananas, almond milk, and vanilla extract. Blend until smooth and creamy.
2. Serve immediately or freeze for 1-2 hours for a firmer texture.

Nutritional Values (per serving):

- Calories: 120 • Protein: 1g • Carbohydrates: 30g • Fat: 1g • Fiber: 3g

Pumpkin Custard

Servings: 4

Cooking Time: 40 minutes

Ingredients

- 1 cup pumpkin puree
- 1/2 cup milk
- 1/4 cup brown sugar
- 1 teaspoon pumpkin pie spice
- 2 eggs

Instructions

1. Preheat oven to 350°F (175°C).
2. In a large bowl, combine pumpkin puree, milk, brown sugar, pumpkin pie spice, and eggs. Mix well.
3. Pour mixture into a greased baking dish.
4. Bake for 35-40 minutes, until custard is set.
5. Serve warm or chilled.

Nutritional Values (per serving):

• Calories: 130 • Protein: 5g • Carbohydrates: 20g • Fat: 4g • Fiber: 2g

Almond Butter Cookies

Servings: 4

Cooking Time: 20 minutes

Ingredients

- 1 cup almond butter
- 1/2 cup sugar
- 1 egg
- 1 teaspoon vanilla extract

Instructions

1. Preheat oven to 350°F (175°C).
2. In a large bowl, combine almond butter, sugar, egg, and vanilla extract. Mix well.
3. Drop by tablespoonfuls onto a greased baking sheet.
4. Bake for 10-12 minutes, until edges are golden brown.
5. Serve warm or at room temperature.

Nutritional Values (per serving):

- Calories: 180 • Protein: 6g • Carbohydrates: 20g • Fat: 10g • Fiber: 3g

Blueberry Crumble

Servings: 4

Cooking Time: 30 minutes

Ingredients

- 2 cups blueberries
- 1/4 cup sugar
- 1/2 cup rolled oats
- 1/4 cup flour
- 1/4 cup brown sugar
- 1/4 cup butter, melted

Instructions

1. Preheat oven to 350°F (175°C).
2. In a large bowl, combine blueberries and sugar. Pour into a greased baking dish.
3. In another bowl, combine oats, flour, brown sugar, and melted butter. Sprinkle over blueberries.
4. Bake for 25-30 minutes, until topping is golden brown.
5. Serve warm.

Nutritional Values (per serving):

• Calories: 200 • Protein: 2g • Carbohydrates: 35g • Fat: 7g • Fiber: 4g

Strawberry Yogurt Bark

Servings: 4

Cooking Time: 15 minutes (plus freezing time)

Ingredients

- 2 cups Greek yogurt
- 1 cup strawberries, sliced
- 2 tablespoons honey

Instructions

1. In a large bowl, mix Greek yogurt and honey.

2. Spread mixture evenly onto a baking sheet lined with parchment paper.

3. Top with sliced strawberries.

4. Freeze for at least 4 hours or until solid.

5. Break into pieces and serve frozen.

Nutritional Values (per serving):

• Calories: 100 • Protein: 5g • Carbohydrates: 15g • Fat: 2g • Fiber: 1g

Pears with Honey and Cinnamon

Servings: 4

Cooking Time: 15 minutes

Ingredients

- 4 pears, halved and cored
- 2 tablespoons honey
- 1/2 teaspoon cinnamon

Instructions

1. Place pear halves on a baking sheet.

2. Drizzle with honey and sprinkle with cinnamon.

3. Bake at 350°F (175°C) for 15 minutes or until tender.

4. Serve warm.

Nutritional Values (per serving):

• Calories: 100 • Protein: 1g • Carbohydrates: 25g • Fat: 0g • Fiber: 4g

Conclusion

Managing gastroparesis through diet can be challenging, but with careful planning and the right recipes, it is possible to maintain a nutritious and enjoyable eating routine. This cookbook has provided a comprehensive guide to understanding gastroparesis and navigating the dietary adjustments necessary for managing this condition.

By following the stages of dietary progression—from liquid and pureed diets to soft solids and maintenance—you can help minimize symptoms and improve your quality of life. The meal plans and recipes included in this book are designed to offer variety, nutritional balance, and ease of preparation, ensuring that you can enjoy your meals while taking care of your digestive health.

Remember, the key to managing gastroparesis is to listen to your body and work closely with your healthcare provider. Each person's experience with gastroparesis is unique, and what works for one person may not work for another. Adjust your diet based on your symptoms and tolerance, and don't hesitate to seek professional advice when needed.

I hope this cookbook has empowered you with the knowledge and tools to take control of your dietary management and enjoy a wide range of delicious and safe foods. Here's to better health and enjoyable eating!

Measurement and Conversions

CUPS	OZ	G	TBSP	TSP	ML
1	8	225	16	48	250
3/4	6	170	12	36	175
2/3	5	140	11	32	150
1/2	4	115	8	24	125
1/3	3	70	5	16	70
1/4	2	60	4	12	60
1/8	1	30	2	6	30
1/16	1/2	15	1	3	15

250°F	300°F	325°F	350°F	400°F	450°F
120°C	150°F	160°C	175°C	200°C	230°C

About the Author

Habeeb Ganiu is a passionate writer about empowering people to lead active healthy lifestyles by teaching them the personalized skills they need to fuel themselves with whole foods while maintaining a healthy life balance.